AF492950

SALUDABLE
MENTE

100 PHYSICAL, MENTAL AND SPIRITUAL HEALTH TIPS

100 PHYSICAL, MENTAL AND SPIRITUAL HEALTH TIPS

Tip 1

Breakfast is the most vital meal. It should not be missed to replenish the body with functional metabolic changes during the long hours of sleep. It is best to include carbohydrates, fats and proteins for ideal nutrition such as combinations of fresh fruits, toast and breakfast cereals with milk.

Tip 2

Maintain a well-balanced diet for a healthy life A well-balanced diet consists of eating different types of nutritious foods in proportion. This will increase your energy and improve your well-being. Excess and deficiency of specific vitamins and minerals can also cause undesirable health effects.

Tip 3

Be aware of the amount of salt you consume during snacks and meals. Table salt is the sodium chloride that is widely used as a flavour enhancer. High sodium intake is a risk factor for diseases such as hypertension, heartburn, osteoporosis and other cardiovascular diseases. Limit your sodium intake by simply reducing your consumption of salty foods without making the choice of salt substitutes.

Tip 4

Stay away from the buffet or "fork free" meals because you may be tempted to eat too much to get a fair value for what you have paid. Otherwise, you may opt for nutritious foods such as fresh fruit, vegetable salads, and low-fat foods. Stand firm and resist the urge to refill your plate a second time.

Tip 5

Limits the intake of processed foods such as canned, refrigerated and dried foods. Food processing alters the natural components of foods, making them less beneficial to the body. The use of chemicals to preserve, control, and enhance flavor can be more harmful to the body's systems than it is to improve health.

Tip 6

Consider eating whole foods. Whole foods are nutritious foods that have their natural compounds intact. They are not processed or refined. They do not contain added chemicals such as flavorings, preservatives, and other ingredients. Start eating whole foods by adding sliced fresh fruits and vegetables to each and every meal.

Tip 7

The best and healthiest way to prepare poultry for a meal is to remove visible skin and fat before cooking. Bake or roast poultry instead of frying it to prevent oil absorption. Between the parts, chicken breasts are high in protein and low in fat, making them the best choice of cuts.

Tip 8

Water is vital for maintaining a healthy life. It is recommended that you drink at least 8 glasses of water every day. It helps cells, tissues and organs function normally. Water deficiency in the body or dehydration can cause serious damage to the kidneys and other organs that can result in mental confusion, coma and even death if intervention is not immediately taken.

Tip 9

Maintain a low-fat diet. Foods that are naturally low in fat are fruits, vegetables, beans and grains. Be sure to check the labels of the products you buy at the market. The label for fat content per serving should be no more than 2-3 grams. It is best to choose a fat content of 1 gram of fat per 100 calories.

Tip 10

Supplement your body with iron nutrition. Iron can only be taken from food sources such as red meat, fish, poultry, cereals, leafy vegetables, and raisins. It serves as fuel to energize our body by assisting in the production of red blood cells. Eat foods rich in iron with vitamin C for effective absorption of iron.

Tip 11

Eating banana for breakfast is an effective weight loss plan known as the Miracle Morning Banana Diet. In this diet plan, all you need is to eat banana for breakfast; drink adequate water; no more eating after 8:00 PM and sleep before midnight. It has been proven to be effective because bananas increase the metabolism.

Tip 12

Include high-fiber foods in your diet plan. It's a simple way to maintain health and fitness. High-fiber foods can be found in whole foods such as fruits, legumes, nuts, grains, and vegetables. Fiber content can help improve your energy and keep you away from diseases like cardiovascular disease.

Tip 13

Carbohydrates don't add weight. It is not advisable to reduce carbohydrate intake because it is the main source of energy and contains little fat. The side dishes that you eat with rice and the spreads that you put on your sandwiches are the ones that should be limited if your goal is to lose weight.

Tip 14

Treat yourself to a fat-free yogurt and combine it with your favorite fruit slices. Dairy products like yogurt are naturally rich in calcium to strengthen bones and in vitamin A which plays a great role in the beauty of our skin. Non-fat yogurt also contains friendly bacteria known as probiotics to improve digestive processes.

Tip 15

Drink orange juice or eat orange every day. Citrus fruits are high in vitamin C, which can enhance our immune system, improving our resistance to infection. It also facilitates the absorption of iron for the prevention of anemia. Other sources of vitamin C are berries, tomatoes, kiwi fruit and green leafy vegetables.

Tip 16

Enjoy eating steamed oysters. Oysters are rich in zinc. Zinc is needed for cell production and tissue repair. It also helps in the normal functioning of the immune system and the reproductive system. Zinc can also be found in other food sources such as beef and pork.

Tip 17

For a brighter, healthier eye, eat foods rich in vitamins A, C, E, beta-carotene and lutein. These are all antioxidants that can decrease the risk of eye problems, especially age-related macular degeneration that can cause blindness as you age. All of these can be taken from green, leafy vegetables.

Tip 18

Don't eat if you're not hungry. It will cause you a lot of weight. When you feel hungry, drink water because sometimes we respond to our thirst by eating. After drinking and still feeling the same, eat but don't overdo it. Do it slowly and enjoy your meal without adding more food to your plate.

Tip 19

Check that you don't eat too much during the holidays. Prepared foods can be very watery, but you should resist it by staying away from preparation. As much as possible, keep in mind that you should only eat nutritious food in a non-excessive amount.

Tip 20

Be aware of what you're drinking. Sodas, coffee, energy drinks, and alcoholic beverages are high in calories. They focus more on increasing the fat in your belly. When you are thirsty, the cheapest and most helpful thing for your body is to drink a glass of water or a freshly squeezed diluted juice.

Tip 21

Junk food literally means useless. It doesn't do your body any good. It's high in sodium, calories and many chemical ingredients to attract shoppers with the artificial flavor. Instead of buying junk food for your snacks and break time, replace it with nutritious fruits and vegetables.

Tip 22

Gradually reduce the sugar in your hot or cold drinks until you no longer need them. White sugar contains no vitamins or minerals, and brown sugar contains a very small amount that is not nutritionally important. Sugar and honey are also fattening and can cause tooth decay.

Tip 23

Give fruit or toys instead of candy and sweets to children as a gift or reward. Children as young associative learners will later associate harmful foods with good events. This may overshadow their thinking about the true value of a healthy, nutritious diet. As much as possible, practice a healthy lifestyle with young people.

Tip 24

It is important to be careful about how much you eat. Know the expected number of servings of packaged food before you eat. Some packaged noodles may be small in packages but are sometimes prepared for two or more people. Others do not realize this and eat the entire package of noodles, causing their calories and food intake to double.

Tip 25

Eat more fish. White fish is low in fat and oily fish is high in omega-3 fatty acids. Fish oil or omega-3 fatty acids are unsaturated oils not found in other food sources. It will help the body fight cholesterol and help maintain healthy heart function.

Tip 26

Omega-3 fatty acids are beneficial for removing cholesterol, but for those who do not like eating oily fish they can be replaced with flax seeds. It is a compound of Omega 3, a fatty acid that is available in different nutrition stores. You can take it once a week as a dietary supplement.

Tip 27

Be careful what you buy at the grocery store, an attractive food package and an expensive price does not necessarily mean it is healthy. Endorsers of famous products can also be very convincing, but you shouldn't believe everything you see and hear from them. It's better to have your own understanding of what's good for you.

Tip 28

The most important thing to know about allergy is the allergen. Allergens are substances that trigger allergy, which can be in the form of dust, pet hair, odours, pollen and smoke. Trace the pattern of your allergy. Sneezing after cleaning the house may mean that the allergens are dust.

Tip 29

Go on an elimination diet if you are suspected of being allergic to food. Do it gradually by eliminating each food you usually eat over a period of 2 to 4 weeks to see the changes. The process will be repeated in reverse order to reintroduce the eliminated food to see if allergic symptoms occur.

Tip 30

The best way to treat food allergy is to avoid its trigger. Check food labels carefully for additives that can cause allergic reactions. If you suspect that a specific additive may cause your allergy, avoid it as much as possible. Consider fresh and unprocessed foods.

Tip 31

Control your food intake by keeping a diary. Make a list of all your activities, including all the foods you eat. Take note when your allergies start to show. You can make a connection between your allergic reactions and a particular food, or something like odors, soap, cosmetics, clothing, or your pet's hair.

Tip 32

Don't hesitate to ask about the ingredients on the menu when you eat at restaurants, parties or when you eat food prepared by someone else. It is important to know this information for your own safety and precaution. Always carry antihistamines or anti-allergy medications prescribed by your doctor with you in case of emergency.

Tip 33

If possible, wear an ID bracelet that indicates your allergy. This will help others know what triggers your allergic reactions in an emergency. You may also consider telling your family, office colleagues and friends about your allergies before you go to a buffet. In this case, they can alert you to the foods you should not eat or drink.

Tip 34

It is important to seek the help of experts such as an allergist or immunologist for a better diagnosis and treatment of your allergies. You can do several tests to identify specific triggers. They will also provide you with a prescription that is right for you.

Tip 35

It is best to check for signs and symptoms of allergies to the widely known food allergens such as soya, milk, peanuts, shellfish and eggs. If they cause itching, sneezing, swelling and hives, keep them away from your home and avoid them as much as possible.

Tip 36

As soon as you discover that you have a food allergy, you should adjust your meal plan as well as your nutritional intake. By getting rid of your food triggers, you may need to supplement the nutrients you have lost. Dietary modifications are necessary, but you should still observe a well-balanced diet to maintain a healthy body without the food triggers.

Tip 37

Sometimes food allergens are your favorite foods, which may be harder to get rid of. Try to condition your mind that the foods and additives that can trigger your allergies are not edible. That way, you can gradually avoid the temptation to eat or taste bites.

Tip 38

It is best not to eat any type of nuts, even if you are aware of the specific type of nut you are allergic to. Determine the contents of what you buy carefully because nuts are not only present in some food products but are also used as ingredients in shampoos, soaps and lotions.

Tip 39

Stress, tension and anxiety can also trigger allergies. Try to determine the causes and address them through relaxation, meditation, reflection, and other types of coping techniques. Drinking milk before bedtime at night can contribute greatly to a good night's rest, thus decreasing your potential to be stressed.

Tip 40

You should always be prepared because allergic reactions can occur at any time and in any place. Imagine beforehand different situations in which you have allergies and how you can handle them if you are away from home. This will help you to prepare and think about your safety first rather than panic and do nothing at all.

Tip 41

If your children have food allergies, teach them not to accept any food given to them by friends, classmates, or anyone else without your confirmation. Let them know what they are allergic to and what symptoms they will show so they can seek help from adults or your school clinic when it happens.

Tip 42

Avoid all types of milk and milk products if you are allergic to milk. Make sure you have alternative nutrition or replace the nutrients in milk by eating foods rich in calcium and vitamin D. Consider eating more spinach and broccoli or talk to a dietitian about a more planned diet.

Tip 43

Supplement your diet with vitamin C. Vitamin C works as a natural anti-allergic. A recommended intake of 1000 mg of vitamin C taken twice a day can be a natural treatment for the relief of your allergies and asthma. It should be taken from fresh citrus fruits, not from canned juices or processed foods.

Tip 44

It is recommended to take a bath before bedtime at night for those with pollen allergies. It is difficult to avoid pollen, but you can reduce your exposure. Stay indoors, especially on hot, dry, and windy days. Always close windows and doors with the air conditioning on.

Tip 45

A carpeted floor is not recommended for people allergic to dust. It will cause continuous sneezing and itching. Otherwise, buy a vacuum cleaner to clean it more often. Bed sheets should also be changed frequently to prevent them from falling. Leaving shoes outside the room is also a good idea to prevent more dust.

Tip 46

It's best not to share your bedroom with your pets, especially if you have allergies. Put them in a separate room to avoid inhaling their hair and dead skin cells. Sometimes, other people who have another type of allergy can develop an allergic reaction to pets more often than those who share a bed with their pets.

Tip 47

Wear gloves and a mask when dusting or cleaning the house to avoid inhaling dust. Store stuffed toys or place them in sealed plastic wrap. Always wash rags off the floor to prevent mold growth. Be sure to vacuum or clean under your bed and always use a damp cloth to remove dust.

Tip 48

For skin allergies such as contact dermatitis, you must know the surface or texture to which you are allergic. The most common causes of skin allergies are fake jewelry, materials made of leather and metals. If you are allergic to these, make sure you put a cloth or cover on them to avoid direct contact with your skin.

Tip 49

Wash the surface of the skin with cold water and mild soap immediately after you have developed a rash and itching from a known chemical irritant. Do not scratch to avoid injury and further infection. You can use calamine lotion to treat itching, but not on the face or near the eyes. If a rash develops continually, seek medical help.

Tip 50

Do a daily exercise or workout routine - Exercise and a daily workout routine will not only give you a healthy body but also help you purify your body and mind by releasing your endorphins and aggressive emotions. Through exercise, you can take in more oxygen allowing your body to pump your blood faster.

Tip 51

Choose to use non-toxic household cleaners - even cleaners that contain toxic chemicals, even if you don't eat them, can enter your body's system through regular use. By using non-toxic cleaners, you can be sure to rid your home of harmful chemicals that may be bad for your health.

Tip 52

Try to stop or at least limit the pills you take daily - although chronic health conditions may result in the need for you to take several types of pills daily, it would be good to try to limit their use as much as possible since simultaneous intake of these pills can result in damage to the kidneys due to their harmful chemical content.

Tip 53

Deep Breathing: Incorporate the habit of deep breathing, especially if you are outdoors, where there is fresh air. Deep breathing can help you to have a relaxed mind and take in much-needed oxygen that can aid in blood circulation.

Tip 54

Eating organic food - today, people are recognizing the importance of organic food in promoting a person's health. By eating lots of fresh, organic fruits and vegetables, the body not only receives harmful chemicals and toxins, but it can also eliminate the toxins you already have in your body.

Tip 55

Limit or stop activities that can cause an unhealthy lifestyle: By stopping gossiping, watching less TV and not having too many activities online, you can have a very restful mind and can start doing more productive and more important activities that won't affect your mood or be harmful to your health instead.

Tip 56

Stop or limit alcohol intake – Since red wine has been shown to be good for the heart due to its resveratrol content, it is still necessary to limit alcohol intake, as too much can result in health and organ damage, e.g. weakening of the heart, liver problems, loss of sleep and feeling of tiredness. You can choose to stop drinking altogether and get resveratrol pills instead.

Tip 57

Apart from those prescribed, it is no secret that dangerous drugs can have many harmful results, some of which are fatal. You can give your body an incredible amount of toxin that can immediately weaken your body's immune system that you need to fight off disease.

Tip 58

Wearing little makeup: Not everyone knows that most makeup available on the market contains chemicals and toxins that can enter the body's system when used. There are many ways to make your makeup look good even if you only use a small amount and know how it will be good for your health. Use makeup that is made of natural or chemical-free ingredients that do not cause you any harm.

Tip 59

Leave your hair alone - if hair sprays can ruin the ozone layer, what else can they do to your own body? The same goes for hair dyes that contain various chemicals with adverse effects on a person's health. Not only will your hair and scalp be affected, but so will your other organs just by breathing in the chemicals they contain.

Tip 60

Have more sex: A good exercise that can have positive results is having sex. Sex can give you more energy, lower cholesterol in your body, increase the flow of oxygen to your brain, help you sleep more, reduce stress and pressure, and even serve as a natural pain reliever.

Tip 61

Juice Fasting - A popular, though controversial, method of detoxification is juice fasting. It is done for the primary purpose of reducing or eliminating cooked food products and animal products that have already accumulated in the body to cleanse the system.

Tip 62

Colon cleansing: Clearly one of the most popular methods of detoxification is colon cleansing. It is the method of cleansing the colon or large intestine of harmful parasites and the bowel that have already accumulated or petrified in the colon, which can lead to poor digestion and disease.

Tip 63

Doing hydrotherapy: This is slowly but surely becoming a popular form of detoxification and is usually offered in saunas and spas. You can also do it in your own home while showering. It is considered one of those alternative methods of detoxification in which the altered water temperature can lead to the body's blood circulation and the removal of waste from the body's tissues.

Tip 64

Brushing the skin: The skin is the largest organ on the body. Therefore, it is most capable of obtaining harmful toxins, allowing toxins to enter your system. By using the detoxification method of skin brushing, the skin is stimulated to remove toxic waste products from your body and makes your kidneys healthier.

Tip 65

Herb intake: Many healthy and natural herbs can play a great role in the body's internal and external detoxification. Examples of these herbs are licorice and cassava roots, which are great laxatives, dandelion and milk thistle for the liver, witch hazel and bilberry, which are good antioxidant and anti-inflammatory herbs, and pumpkin seeds, which can rid the body of parasites.

Tip 66

Meditation is a great way to detoxify the mind and body from poisonous energy and thought drains that can be very harmful. Choose the best meditation guides available and follow a specific schedule and program that you can do regularly.

Tip 67

Do the meditation alone: Doing the meditation alone is the most effective way to do it if you want to get immediate results. To do it well, you must eliminate any discomfort or inconvenience that could ruin your concentration. Use a comfortable place with the right lighting and temperature. Be patient with the results as they do not happen overnight.

Tip 68

De-stress through various effective methods: There are many ways to get rid of stress and pressure, such as getting counselling. Be open to being more sociable, do activities that can improve self-confidence and set realistic goals. By understanding and being happy with your body, you shouldn't have to feel insecure about doing things that can be harmful to your body.

Tip 69

Eat plenty of fiber: It is already known that eating foods with fiber can greatly help cleanse the body's digestive tract of various toxins and accumulated feces. Some of the best foods with fiber are brown rice, broccoli, wheat bread, corn, bran cereal, and, of course, fruits and vegetables.

Tip 70

Drink plenty of water: It is easily one of the most effective and inexpensive ways to cleanse your system and eliminate toxins. Drinking water is much healthier than drinking soda, alcohol or juice when you are thirsty or after a meal. Try to discipline yourself to only drink water.

Tip 71

Don't eat junk food: Junk food may be easy and tasty to eat, but it's processed, which means it contains chemicals and sweeteners and unnatural flavors that can easily bring poison and toxins into your system. Not only can junk food have adverse and unhealthy effects on you, but it can also make you overweight.

Tip 72

Eating Raw Foods: There are many raw food and raw food detox diet that are effective in detoxifying your body. They can help cleanse your body of processed ingredients and animal products that have already built up in your system.

Tip 73

Eat healthy antioxidant foods: There are many types of foods and nutrients that you can eat or drink to help with detoxification, cranberries that promote sharp brains and is a great antioxidant, vitamin C, is a perfect detoxification agent for the liver because of its glutathione content and garlic which is also rich in antioxidants and a known ingredient for health purposes.

Tip 74

Eat organic, locally grown, and ethical foods: By including organic foods in your daily diet, as well as locally grown foods that are sure to be free of pesticides, you can be sure to not only make your body healthy and free of toxins, but also help your community. So by eating ethical foods you will ensure that those foods do not come from slaughterhouses, etc.

Tip 75

Yoga is easily one of the favorite options for exercises that can eliminate stress and toxin in the body, facilitating the mind, promoting breathing, lowering blood pressure, improving rest and sleep, promoting better digestion, and improving posture and concentration.

Tip 76

Cardiovascular exercise: This type of exercise can easily promote health and is a great workout for replenishing calories. A scheduled cardio workout can also be good for anger management, resulting in a more relaxed body and mind.

Tip 77

Regular swimming exercises: Now considered a good detoxification exercise as it works the heart and muscles and promotes better breathing and gives a better body temperature, thus helping the internal cleansing of the body. However, it would be better to swim in a pool with natural water rather than chlorinated water.

Tip 78

Attend Pilates classes: This is another workout, like yoga, that will not only increase your energy, but also promote your immune system that won't even require you to have cardiovascular exercises that will induce sweating from your body. Like yoga, it is also a very popular workout today, even for celebrities.

Tip 79

Do exercises that reduce fat and make you sweat. These exercises will not only give you a well-toned and better-formed body, but will also cleanse you of toxins stored and located on the surface of the body. You need to know which are the right exercises that will make you sweat and lose unhealthy fat.

Tip 80

Exercise for a good night's sleep: Since proper sleep is necessary to eliminate toxins from your system, the ideal would be to do the right exercise that induces you to sleep well and peacefully. Make this a habit and make sure you protect your sleep environment from distractions such as the TV, computer, or too many lights.

Tip 81

Have a lifestyle that is holistic: To have a holistic lifestyle is to live a life that takes into account the health of body, mind and spirit, all at the same time and not just one of them. In this way, you can control not only your health but also the toxicity of your body in its entirety and not just in part.

Tip 82

Avoiding promiscuity: By living a life free of perversion and promiscuity, you will not only avoid suffering the emotional drain that these actions can bring, but you will also avoid possible diseases and problems caused by these acts of perversion such as STDs and other sexually related diseases or, even worse, AIDS.

Tip 83

Proper hygiene: Hygiene affects a person's overall health and keeps toxins out of your body. Make sure you always bathe at least once a day and make sure you brush and floss your teeth several times a day, preferably after every meal. Also, wash your hands as often as possible, especially before you eat.

Tip 84

Being a vegetarian: Although it's difficult for many people who have become accustomed to eating meat, vegetarians out there are enjoying the benefits of not eating red meat, chicken, or any other animal food. Vegetables and fruits have always been associated with good nutrients needed to cleanse the system. They can even help the environment in the process.

Tip 85

Having a macrobiotic lifestyle: Having a life like this means that you will live based on the harmony of your life with nature by having a good lifestyle and proper diet combined with your love and respect for the environment. There are many ways to do this, especially today when people are becoming very aware of the environmental problems we are experiencing.

Tip 86

Having a therapeutic and strategic body massage: By obtaining the services of someone who can give you such a massage, you will be able to enjoy its benefits such as a better digestive system and the stimulation of your body's ability to get rid of waste.

Tip 87

Use a car that is environmentally friendly: Getting rid of environmental pollutants is one way to eliminate toxins that can enter your body. If you use a car that doesn't generate more pollution, such as an electric car or one that runs on water, that you and your loved one can breathe easily, you can reduce the amount of toxic gases in the air.

Tip 88

Growing houseplants: Doing this will not only make your house look more beautiful, but will also allow oxygen to flow freely in your environment, allowing you to take in enough, which will promote your breathing, as well as purify the air by preventing the production of more carbon dioxide, which could be harmful.

Tip 89

Proper composting and disposal of pet waste, along with a healthy body, should be a healthy environment. Since garbage is a part of life and pets are a common fixture in many homes, proper disposal of pet waste and garbage is necessary. Composting or recycling garbage or using it to enrich your yard is good advice.

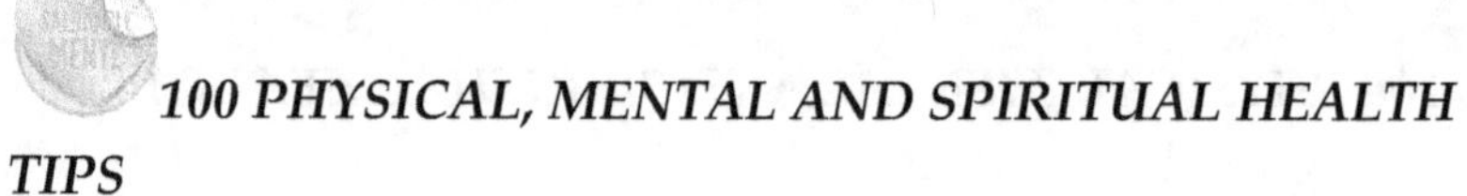

Tip 90

Grow a garden: Speaking of gardens, having a home with a garden will give its inhabitants a complete and continuous supply of oxygen that is needed in various body systems. It is also good to grow fruits and vegetables in the garden itself that can be used at home.

Tip 91

Adequate air supply: Air is important to your health and your system. Make sure there is more than enough of it in your home by having adequate ventilation in your rooms and regularly changing air filters and making use of carpets and furniture made of natural materials.

Tip 92

Use Aromatherapy: There are now many of these aromatherapy methods available on the market, including the Internet. Most of these products work as promised and are great techniques to help cure certain ailments and colds as well as relieve stress.

Tip 93

Don't let work stress you out. For some people, their job is a form of stress, something they can't wait to do but do every day for a living. This shouldn't be the case. Instead, you should learn to enjoy your work or at least make it acceptable by being more organized and avoiding annoying co-workers.

Tip 94

Knowing when to stop paying attention: By learning to stop paying attention, you can give your mind and body the proper rest they need, particularly from your gossipy co-workers and friends, from your e-mails or Twitter messages, or from anything that happens around you that might give you unnecessary excitement or even irritation.

Tip 95

Learn to say "NO": You can say "NO" to anything you think will only cause you harm, such as eating bad food, drinking alcohol, doing stressful events, losing sleep over something, and anything else that is stressful and will only lead to an unhealthy lifestyle. Saying NO to this will do you good.

Tip 96

Lead a simple life: By doing this, you can focus more on keeping your body and your lifestyle healthy. The more you do, the less time you have to think about things that make you aware of the harmful toxins and chemicals in the environment that can harm you. However, if you do it simply, you will also have time for yourself.

Tip 97

Learn to maintain what you have already achieved: Having a healthy and adequate diet is already difficult. Even more difficult is the task of maintaining it and making sure that what you have previously achieved in terms of health and detoxification is not wasted by simply returning to your bad habits.

Tip 98

Leave the couch and get on with your healthy lifestyle: Remember that resisting the temptation to sit on the couch all day means fighting the temptation of the main culprits of obesity, such as overeating (especially junk food), oversleeping and, of course, the unhealthy sedentary lifestyle.

Tip 99

Make your exercise or fitness regimen fun and interesting by including other people in your daily routine. For example, take a walk in the park with your adorable dog or go jogging every morning with your best friend. In some cases, join exercise groups to make new friends and get more exercise tips.

Tip 100

Choose an exercise or fitness regimen that you know you can handle. Not every exercise works for everyone. So be sure to do your research first, especially if you are thinking about a new exercise program. Talk to your body and see how far you think your system can go before deciding what fitness program to follow.

I hope these 100 health tips have helped you a lot! Success and prosperity!

www.ingramcontent.com/pod-product-compliance
Lightning Source LLC
Chambersburg PA
CBHW072020150726
47999CB00002B/737